WEIGHTED

Understanding The True Burden of Your
Unmet Needs And How That Affects
Your Weight Loss

Zen Burgos

Title: Weighted: Understanding The True Burden of Your Unmet Needs And How That Affects Your Weight Loss

By: Zen Burgos

ISBN for Print: 979-8-9892139-1-7

Cover design: Rhianon Paige

Editing: Dustin Dixon

Published by: AFGO Press

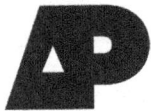

Printed in the United States

First Edition 2023

For Chariot

*May you grow up knowing you deserve to have
all your wounds healed.*

I love you forever and always.

TABLE OF CONTENTS

BEFORE WE GET STARTED...

Dear Reader,

In the coming pages, I will refer to a process that I call the "Healthy Freedom Formula" and I'll explain how it changed my life by combining my decades of fitness and nutrition expertise with the tools I learned while healing from emotionally painful experiences from my past. Some of those experiences were pushed so deep down into my unconscious mind that I never realized I had been self-sabotaging for decades.

My hope is that my Healthy Freedom Formula™ will also help you feel more confident, healthy, energized and free from those heavy burdens you might not even realize you've been carrying.

To better understand what may be getting in the way of not only your weight loss efforts but the limitless version of yourself and your life, I invite you to go to www.zenburgos.com and download my **WEIGHTED Quiz** to see how "weighted" you are. It's free, and it may turn out to be the start of your very own en*lightening* transformation.

Health & Happiness,
-Zen

INTRODUCTION

What the F%#k Is Wrong With You People?

"Would you like to meet your granddaughter?" I asked my mom while I held my baby out to her.

"I can see her from here," she replied, leaning on a chair across the room.

My mom refused to even hold my child.

My father then walked over to hold her and told me she was beautiful. He didn't even question my mother's behavior, which was typical.

Thankfully, I hadn't married a man who even closely resembled my father.

My husband's reaction?

"What the fuck is wrong with you people?!"

It turns out that there was a lot "wrong" with them, but it used to look "normal" to me. It's how I grew up. I thought that's just the way parents were. But it wasn't until that day in my sister's living room, as I offered them what I thought would be a highlight of their lives – to hold their brand new grandchild – that I realized just how messed up my parents were.

My brother, who lived in Los Angeles, had always preached, "Don't get sucked into the crazy." But I didn't realize he was talking about our family until then.

On the other hand, my sister couldn't understand why it would bother me that *my own mother* wouldn't want to hold *my newborn baby.*

My husband was right. *What the fuck was wrong with these people?*

In the year following the birth of my daughter, there was lots of stress eating and a few more failed attempts at holiday get-togethers, which I felt obligated to attend. My parents either ignored me completely or if they did talk to me, it was as if I were some stranger asking for directions.

Out of the blue, my sister suggested we all see her therapist together.

My sister had a therapist? The sister who would never acknowledge or validate my feelings? The sister who had me believe there was nothing wrong with our family?

The sister that made me believe it was *just me?*

While setting up that appointment, her therapist told me,

"There's no worse position than being in the middle like your sister."

I couldn't take it. I had to push back. "Excuse me. You're totally invalidating my position. I think it's harder to be ignored by one's parents completely after moving across the country to be closer to them and after having a new baby!"

She apologized.

And then, after meeting with all of us over several sessions, I asked the therapist if she thought there was a good reason for my parents to treat me this way.

She said, "No, absolutely not. Unfortunately, your parents... especially your mother... are very stuck in their ways, and it's not likely they will ever change."

Later, I got my own therapist, who explained that "stuck in their ways" was a nice way of saying my parents were "emotionally immature" and not likely to evolve at this point.

She also told me something that would change my life forever: "Not only did you never deserve to be treated like that... but you do not want your daughter thinking those are safe people to be around."

BAM!

That's what it took for me to break the chain of trauma in my family. I was going to protect my daughter at all costs.

My therapist's words became permanently planted in my head.

Those words set me free.

They would guide me forever more.

Now, the work of becoming the woman I was meant to be could begin.

I began seeking healthier coping mechanisms to undo all the harmful effects of living with an emotionally abusive family. Stress eating was NOT a healthy coping mechanism. I was still far from healing - but I was at least aware now that something needed to change.

I knew my pain was valid – but it was a while until I realized how much invalidating my pain for so many years was affecting my body despite my nutrition and exercise expertise. My coping mechanisms sabotaged my weight loss efforts as well as my potential in other areas of my life – and I never realized how much until after having my baby in my forties.

My physical, emotional, and mental potential had been *weighted* down for decades, and I didn't even know it.

I'm using the word "weighted" to identify the symptom of unconsciously carrying the burdens caused by unmet needs that began in childhood and continued into adulthood.

Emotionally, our unhealed traumas are weighing us down, and for many of us, that also equals body fat weighing us down. I want you to think of it as a heavy weight you can remove – just like you can take off a backpack full of rocks. Those burdens you're dealing with, those unhealed traumas, and those unhealthy coping mechanisms are not who you are.

For me, all that unhealed trauma was like carrying around a 40-pound bowling ball… and it showed up on my body as extra fat. It showed up as having a lack of boundaries because I had put others' emotional needs before my own for so long. It showed up as devaluing myself and my opinions in so many relationships and failed businesses.

It was so much more than just needing to lose some weight.

I was constantly overindulging in unhealthy behaviors to soothe myself, like eating sugar, Netflix marathons, or playing games, because I was ***emotionally starved*** for the love, comfort, and acceptance I craved from my parents. I was allowing my coping mechanisms to sabotage my potential. And I had sabotaged myself for DECADES.

I realized that achieving great health is like piecing together a unique puzzle that combines not only nutrition and exercise needs but also takes into account genetics, past experiences, subconscious beliefs, and coping mechanisms.

Your coping mechanisms are strategies that impact not only your health but also your work, your relationships, and your confidence.

If your coping mechanisms sabotage those important aspects of your life, you're not going to make progress.

That truth, my friend, is why your diet and exercise regimen doesn't work. Or why you can't seem to live your best life when it comes to your body, your job, or your relationships.

The good news is that you can mend all those puzzle pieces and combine them to create your best life once you become aware of the issues and find the right strategies to heal your body and reprogram your mind.

That's how I discovered my Healthy Freedom Formula. It takes you through four steps to get you to a place where you feel confident, healthy, energized, and free from those chains you didn't even realize were holding you back from a more fulfilling life. It is a formula that is weighted in your favor (nice for once, right?!) and designed to give you and your body the advantage you have needed for so long.

Of course, it's essential to move and eat in an efficient and healthy way for weight loss, but the first step in my Healthy Freedom Formula is WEIGHTED AWARENESS, where you give yourself the gift of your full attention – to examine your unhealthy habits to see how, when, and why you adopted them and how they have become an invisible weight that you carry around every minute of every day.

What emotional issues have been weighing you down that physically "weighted" you beyond where you'd like to be?

Lasting weight loss is not just sticking to a diet and exercise plan. It's seeing why you adopt certain behaviors when you go "off plan."

Let's face it, anyone can go for walks and eat chicken on a salad for thirty days and lose weight, but to keep it off takes a different approach. It helps to look into WHY you grab WHAT you grab when you finally binge after an unsustainable thirty days of being "good."

While growing up, we all adopt strategies for dealing with the world. Perhaps you've been eating treats at night to reward yourself for getting through the day. Maybe a glass of wine (or two) has become your daily relaxing ritual.

Maybe you eat more on the weekend because you keep meaning to start your diet on Monday. Maybe you scroll on your phone a little too much.

Maybe you hold your tongue to keep the peace instead of speaking your mind in a respectful way. Perhaps you always put others before yourself.

Maybe you stay at an unfulfilling job or a relationship because the alternative feels scary. Perhaps you raise your voice or get physical when you're frustrated. Maybe you keep to yourself because people have let you down so much.

You may even feel bad about yourself after you choose some of these strategies.

The reality is that these behaviors are often symptoms of an overarching problem: Emotional Starvation.

Some strategies are healthier and more effective than others, and you shouldn't berate yourself for doing the best you could with the information you had at the time. But suppose some of your strategies for dealing with the world include behavior that makes you feel sick, angry, cruel, poor, or isolated. In that case, you might want to consider upgrading your strategies to healthier options.

For example, some of the strategies you used may have been due to how you chose to deal with trauma or unmet needs and didn't even realize it at the time. You might STILL be invalidating your own pain from your past - which is keeping you in an unhealthy cycle.

Becoming aware of your pain – and validating it – is a crucial first step toward healing disempowering behaviors that keep you overweight, unfulfilled, and unhappy.

Also, 95% of your feel-good neurotransmitters are made in your gut, so if you're inflamed around your belly, chances are you're not feeling as good as you should because your body can't produce the normal level of serotonin if inflammation is impeding that process. Can you see how this situation could create a downward spiral for your motivation?

When I was depressed, I didn't feel like working out. Plus, when I finally forced myself to exercise, my knees and my back would hurt, and I'd be sore for days. But lack of exercise also means a lack of resilience when it comes to stress-induced depression. It's no secret that exercise can elevate mood, but it wasn't until recently that "hope molecules" were discovered to be released when muscles contract.

I'll get more into this later, but I think you can see how awareness of your coping strategies, inflammation in the body, and lack of exercise can produce a not-so-ideal situation when it comes to weight loss and your confidence level.

Step 2 in the Healthy Freedom Formula is WEIGHTED ACCEPTANCE.

After you've become aware that some strategy you adopted made you feel (literally and figuratively) heavy – it's time to look at the consequences. I encourage you to accept this is where you are, right now, today, without arguing against what is. Don't try to soften the blow to yourself in some way.

You've done that for too long. You got here because this is all you knew. You're about to know better so you can do better.

Everything you've learned about your health, your body, and how you feel about yourself was programmed into you, willingly or otherwise.

You knew no other way. As a result, you tried to come up with ways to feel better. Food is an obvious choice for so many people, but there's also alcohol, smoking, gaming, sex, overspending, and a million other ways of distracting yourself from the pain you are in.

Weighted acceptance is not just seeing the negative consequences of your vices but accepting and loving yourself despite using those strategies or coping mechanisms.

Step 3 is all about WEIGHTLESS RESPONSIBILITY.

As a victim of childhood trauma, I would never say that anyone is responsible for their traumatizing event(s). Neither can we blame ourselves for all the ways we tried to cope without really knowing what we were dealing with.

Taking responsibility means we step into our new role as the only authority figure in our life and decide from there what the best course of action will be. Healing how you think about those past hurts (which you absolutely can do) and utilizing new strategies will make you better able to respond in healthier ways and improve your "response-ability."

Step 4 is when we're finally free to take WEIGHTLESS INSPIRED ACTION.

Now that you're aware of the problem, why you have it, how you were not to blame, and how it is your responsibility to solve the problem, you've earned the right to take action in a way that feels motivating and inspiring — no more futile attempts to be healthy while fighting a battle in your subconscious mind.

How is my Healthy Freedom Formula different from everything else you've tried?

First of all, it's weighted in your favor, not in favor of another new diet designed to make money for the "next best greatest diet." If you're anything like me, you've tried just about every diet out there: Weight Watchers, Paleo, Atkins, Keto... and they didn't work.

Why?

Because they only teach you how to DO things (i.e., how to eat and how to exercise) without first changing the way you think about WHY you're comforting yourself with pizza or a margarita.

It's not about what you eat; it's about how you handle life's stressors using old trauma responses that sabotage every effort to make any diet work.

In other words, you're doomed from the start unless you take an entirely different approach to freeing your body from extra weight and old wounds that have remained unhealed.

I've taken my decades of fitness and nutrition coaching experience and combined it with the best self-development and healing techniques that I've found to help you produce the quickest and longest-lasting results in a non-judgy way. I don't know about you, but I always felt like I couldn't admit to eating a box of Reese's to my trainer after a bad day. I knew it was wrong. I knew they'd give me shit about it. So I wouldn't say anything. But looking at that behavior is where the GOLD is! That's where you can learn so much about your stress response, and then you can work on CHANGING it.

I've found no other program that combines all of the necessary elements (and in the correct order!) to change your life by healing those unhealthy coping strategies BEFORE getting to the most effective nutrition and exercises for weight loss.

What's truly unique about my Healthy Freedom Formula is that it provides you with a step-by-step system to help you overcome metabolic challenges, heal from past experiences, and identify subconscious (self-sabotaging) beliefs and harmful coping mechanisms with targeted changes to your nutrition, exercise, psychology, and lifestyle.

The choice to change is yours.

You can choose to stay in the painful situation you're in. (And let's face it, without making changes now, it's probably going to get worse.) Or you can try a new approach to weight loss by examining your unconscious and unhealthy habits to transform your life.

I wish I had the guidance and courage to change decades ago, but I didn't know any better and I didn't have the tools. I weep for the years of pain and frustration I could have avoided, but more than that, I regret missing out on what my life could have been had I validated my pain and utilized healthier coping mechanisms.

Dean Graziosi, a mentor of mine, shared a powerful image with me. He said, "Imagine you're at the end of your life, and you meet God. He holds up an iPhone to show you a video of what your life COULD HAVE BEEN had you not played it small. You see all your unfulfilled dreams and potential right there in front of you, and you BEG to go back and try it again... but you can't because now it's too late."

That story really struck me, and I don't want to have regrets like that. I already have so many. Now that I know better, I'm not going to let something as fixable as nutrition, exercise, and healing unmet needs hold me back. And with my help, neither will you.

You CAN wake up happy and excited to start your day. You CAN feel confident and energized in a strong and healthy body. You CAN feel peaceful and supported in your relationships and your work.

You CAN love yourself and your life completely.

But without a mind/body approach, things are more likely to get worse. And it's not as simple as, "eat less, move more."

You and I both know there is much more to it than that.

Without this mind/body approach, lasting weight loss will likely be forever elusive, and you'll continue hurting. When you stay stuck in your emotional pain, your body will continue to physically ache as your body cries, "I'm hurting! I need comfort! I need to be acknowledged!" That little voice inside you is your soul screaming for change, love, support, and acceptance... not potato chips.

I invite you to begin examining how you've been secretly sabotaging yourself **right now**.

In the next chapter, I'll share with you what I discovered in my own journey and how it applies to you as well.

THE HEALTHY
FREEDOM FORMULA

After discovering the truth about my parents, my life began to change.

Finally, I had some answers, validation, and support. But man… I had some Nutella, too — lots of it.

I stopped looking at the scale after I was over 200 pounds. I knew it wasn't good to fixate on a number, but I also knew I needed to make changes.

I'm talking about the kind of changes that are weighted with meaning and purpose. After all, what did it matter if I weighed 200 pounds or 120 pounds… misery doesn't discriminate according to weight. I wanted to find my way to "Healthy Freedom" in my mind so that my body could figure out how much it actually needed to weigh.

At 42 years old, I had a wonderful husband and a healthy baby girl. We got a new house and got our puppy back. There was a lot to be grateful for.

And yet, I still had obsessive, sad thoughts about my parents. I replayed situations in my head, constantly trying to change the outcome.

What did I do that was so wrong? Why were they treating me this way? How could they be so cruel and so hurtful?

I would NEVER treat my daughter the way they were treating me. That was the worst I had ever felt in my life, just when I should have been the happiest.

I ate full King Size Hershey bars at least once a day.

I ate whatever I wanted, actually, because while breastfeeding, you're told not to eat any "diet" food because it's bad for the baby.

So, while I ate a lot of nutritious food for HER, I justified eating a lot of "bad food" for ME. It was the first time in decades that I had REAL Coke instead of Diet.

I had full cheeseburgers WITH THE BUN. I ate all the carbs along with lots of vegetables.

Little did I know that these cravings really stemmed from the fact that I was emotionally starving in so many areas of my life.

And my husband, bless his heart, would get all of that junk for me. He lovingly calls himself "The Enabler." All he knew was that yummy food made me happier in the moment, and my husband wanted to make me happy. But I knew that if my weight continued to increase, I was not going to be happy... or healthy. I needed changes.

I went back to my old standby. I was going to teach group fitness until I got back in shape. That worked for me before, so I thought I'd do that again. I was hired at a big box gym and taught some step, lifting, and cycling classes. I was feeling better, and my weight came down a bit, but I was still addicted to sugar. I saw my therapist regularly, and talk therapy made me feel better, but it wasn't solving my physical health problems or emotional eating. What was really infuriating was that exercise and nutrition techniques that worked before didn't work the same in my 40s. Some of what I did actually made the problem worse.

"Just eat less and move more," they said. Bah! There are only so many calories you can cut before your body rebels from that strategy. My weight problem was not simply about calories. Little did I know this was just the start of my awareness-building journey.

With the financial support of a dear friend, a couple of years later, I was able to open a group fitness studio in my hometown of LaGrange, IL, that combined ellipticals and strength training for people like me who had bad knees and needed nutritional guidance for weight loss.

I felt like if I could just get this business up and running, I could share this new method with the world and help people like me, and THEN I would feel worthy. After the first year in business, I finally got back down to my pre-pregnancy weight! My studio won awards, and the community seemed to love it – until the pandemic hit and 80% of my membership got Pelotons, and I had to close the studio forever at the end of December 2021.

What I didn't see was that my business had provided a level of "high" for me that food used to give me. In other words, something outside of me was responsible for making me happy.

That's when I really hit rock bottom. My health was at an all-time low. The stress of trying to keep the business open and pay all the bills while little money was coming in was too much.

I couldn't sleep. I had pains everywhere in my body. I felt so much shame for not being able to make this business work despite other gyms being able to keep their doors open. I had sacrificed so much time, money, and energy to try to make this business work – and I felt so much guilt for being away from my girl during those early years.

I couldn't get those back, and now I had nothing to show for it either, except a ton of debt from trying to keep the business afloat. I told myself that I needed to stop working completely and take a break, or the business would kill me.

I stopped answering any phone calls. I disappeared from social media. I imagined my competitors and my parents rejoicing in my failure. (My parents never tried to reach out or come into the studio even though it was 5 minutes from their home.)

All I wanted to do was cocoon with my daughter and my husband and try and get back some of that lost time - which of course, we can't do, but I tried. I sat on the couch, watched Netflix, and ate every comforting thing I could. I went outside for occasional walks, but that was it. I started getting headaches, pains in my abdomen and back, and shooting pains down my legs, knees, and heels. Everything ached.

I knew my mental state was affecting my body. I knew my body was affecting my mental state, too. I knew a lot. But it wasn't enough. I needed more help than I was getting. I reached out for therapy again since that helped me get out of the crisis before.

It's expensive to try to get healthy after hitting rock bottom. I think most doctors only treat your symptoms instead of getting to the root of your disease.

Plus, doctors can make mistakes. In my case, I know I developed knee pain twenty years earlier after a doctor prescribed ciprofloxacin for a bladder infection, and it inflicted permanent damage to my knees.

I didn't have back pain until I visited a chiropractor for the first time for a "preventative wellness adjustment" over eighteen years prior. He failed to see my spondylolisthesis on the X-ray before cracking my back – and severely injured my spine.

The only fix for me now is spinal surgery, but I intend to put that off forever if I can. I should have sued these doctors for the pain and loss of YEARS of work (I couldn't function properly as a personal trainer), but I didn't value myself enough to do that at the time. It makes me angry when I think about it. But in this life, it's "live and learn."

I didn't value myself. And there was nothing and no one in the world that could fix that but me.

Now, I had to learn how to heal myself mentally and physically. I used to think that everything was "fixable," but now I realize that some issues are irreversible IF you let them get to the point of no return.

Some relationships are broken forever. Surgeries can only do so much. If you let fear keep you from doing those things you want to do in life, you've only got so much time – and then that's it.

I decided that I would tackle all aspects of healing: mental, emotional, and physical. I read books, followed specialists, and met with therapists. I worked with conventional doctors as well as alternative healers. I got a coach to keep me accountable with an exercise and nutrition program. I got lab work done and tried new medications and supplements.

It was at this point that my **Healthy Freedom Formula** began to emerge.

Therapy helped my mental state… but didn't fix my cravings.

Workouts helped me boost my metabolism and mood for a bit… but not enough to compensate for emotional eating.

Nutritional support helped my digestion and immune system… but my sleep and hormones suffered without healthy coping techniques.

Medications would help some things, but some had side effects that caused other problems.

Business coaching gurus promised me results, but without all the rest in place, I didn't value myself and made financial decisions based on a feeling of scarcity and a lack of confidence.

I realized that I had to implement ALL of these aspects of healing, and in the right order, to finally turn my life around and break free from the shackles of my generational trauma, bad habits, and perceived limitations.

Unmet Needs

So, the main problem I found was that I had unmet needs as a child. Having unmet needs, in my case, manifested as self-soothing behavior, which included emotional eating and cravings, as well as having a lack of boundaries and doubting myself in my relationships and in my work. Additionally, some medications I had taken in the past had destroyed my gut health, which caused a massive imbalance and disease in my body when combined with my emotional distress.

Once again, symptoms of Emotional Starvation had led to a number of severe consequences in my life.

I was eating food to gain a small measure of comfort that was lacking in the other areas. Starving emotionally, especially as a child, can have long-reaching effects throughout a person's life.

I learned that this happens when you grow up accustomed to erratic and emotionally immature behavior from your caregivers. You think it's normal, and you learn to expect it. Not only that, but you believe if YOU could only be smart enough, strong enough, helpful enough, or funny enough (pick any ___ "enough"), they would love you the way you need to be loved. You blame yourself. You spend your life devaluing yourself, your opinions, and your needs because you were conditioned to believe that you don't matter as much as everyone else.

You're also doomed to repeat this cycle with your own children unless you do some specific things to heal it. This cycle is one form of generational trauma.

Oh, and here's the other thing... even if your parents are AMAZING, they're still only human and will still make mistakes and cannot meet all your needs all the time. So even if you're saying to yourself, "Huh, my childhood was pretty good, actually…" but you're still having trouble with emotional eating or lack of confidence, I guarantee you've got some unmet needs that need addressing. Perhaps you've also had some toxic exposure, medication, or injury that caused some imbalance in your body.

It's not your fault that you don't know what you don't know.

That's why step one is Weighted Awareness.

Do you have any "soft addictions" to help you deal with uncomfortable thoughts or feelings? Soft addictions are typically socially acceptable forms of self-soothing behavior like after-dinner snacks, daily desserts, drinking alcohol nightly or excessively socially, Netflix marathons, frequent online shopping, playing games on your devices to avoid work or responsibilities, excessive exercise, etc.

Has your body weight increased after a particularly stressful time in your life?

Do you feel stuck in your relationships or work?

If you answered yes to any of these questions, then you have at least one emotional puzzle piece of pain that needs mending.

Is your belly puffy? Do you have constant body aches? Have you worked harder than ever and still see the number on the scale increase? Or maybe you stopped exercising altogether because it hurts too much?

If you answer yes to any of those questions, you have at least one crucial physical aspect of your body that needs addressing. Your current nutrition and exercise plan isn't serving you, and it needs to work WITH your current lifestyle and capabilities.

Step Two is Weighted Acceptance.

Humans are wired to be more motivated to get away from pain than we are to go toward pleasure. I had to accept that I had been using unhealthy coping strategies for too long to mask emotional and physical pain - and that my coping strategies were not working to improve my life.

If you get sliced open with a knife, a shot of morphine will make you feel better – but unless you stop the bleeding and heal the wound… you're going to die.

Similarly, overindulging will never be the cure for our emotional starvation.

Step Three is Weightless Responsibility.

It's no one else's choice if I choose to eat or drink substances that can inflame and debilitate my body. We also have the power to choose what thoughts we focus on. We have the ability to learn new strategies that empower us.

If you choose NOT to learn new strategies that can help you, then you'll stay stuck where you're at, and you've got no one else to blame. Once you became an adult, the responsibility to heal yourself became all yours. Life will be more tedious, frustrating, painful, and shorter than it could be unless you choose to take responsibility for your body and your life. However, once you learn these new strategies, your ability to respond to triggers in an empowered way increases dramatically.

Step 4 is Weightless Inspired Action.

There are a number of healing modalities out there, and I've personally tried many that didn't work and had a lot of out-of-pocket expenses. I've made my physical and mental health a priority, so I've devoted tens of thousands of dollars toward my healing. But just because something's expensive doesn't mean it's going to help.

Some techniques took just a few minutes to neutralize a Reese's Peanut Butter Cup craving and helped me more than 12-week programs. Another method I tried took just a couple of hours and released some heel pain I'd had for decades. Another strategy helped me feel more peaceful and supported in just one session than I did with months of therapy.

If you aim to feel more confident, healthy, energized, and free in your body, you've come to the right place. If you're ready to do away with unhealthy coping mechanisms and get to the bottom of why you have them in the first place, then the Healthy Freedom Formula is for you. You won't need to spend tens of thousands of dollars like I did. But you will have to follow the steps exactly, or you'll miss a crucial part of your healing that builds a foundation for the next step.

Digging into your unmet needs can be difficult and messy, and by the way, EVERYONE has unmet needs from childhood – it's just that some of us have more than others. If you stop while you're in that part of the process without getting through it, you'll be stuck in your pain. But don't worry... that's why I'm here to guide you through it. We don't want you to continue to blame someone else for your unmet needs. There's no power in that. Besides, blame at this stage only results in self-sabotage, and I'm guessing you're tired of that, too.

I want to show you why it's important that you can now, years later, heal that unmet need, even from childhood, and heal those unhealthy coping mechanisms that went right along beside it. Once you do that, your exercise and nutrition will be so much easier to dial in.

Take my client Aubrey (name changed to protect her privacy), a successful business owner in Los Angeles. Her weight had fluctuated for quite a few years and she was beating herself up over being unable to stick with a diet or consistently workout. Her weight seemed to increase even when she thought she was being "good." And weight loss had gotten significantly harder after she turned forty, too.

As a trainer, I had helped her increase her muscle mass and lose some body fat years before, but when I moved back to Chicago and stopped training together, her weight went back on. We kept in touch as friends through the pandemic, and I shared my struggles and journey with her. I asked her if I could guide her through some of the neuroscience techniques I had discovered to see if they helped.

Surprisingly, after just a few minutes of questioning, we found a connection between her childhood and her current emotional eating behaviors. She remembered that the only time she and her dad had quality time together was when they would walk to a cafe and get various treats, like cookies. She felt like she had to hide things from her mom, so she never ate treats in front of her mother. After talking Aubrey through some visualization exercises for a few minutes, I asked her how she felt. She laughed and said, "I don't know if it's a coincidence or not... but I don't want cookies anymore."

Wouldn't it be great to not rely on willpower and struggle for weight loss? Wouldn't it be great to just NOT WANT THE COOKIES ANYMORE?

If you're ready to heal, let's dive deeper into the first step in the next chapter: WEIGHTED AWARENESS.

STEP 1

Weighted Awareness

Step 1 in the Healthy Freedom Formula is about Weighted Awareness because you have to know you've got an issue first before you can work on it, like shining your flashlight upon a treasure chest in the darkness. Seeing where the connections are between your self-soothing behaviors and your unmet needs is GOLD, baby!

Once you are aware of those connections causing your compulsive behavior, you can begin the process of changing your life by removing those "heavy weights" (a.k.a. unhealed traumas and unmet needs) that have weighted you down.

After talking to so many people about their struggles with weight loss, I've found one huge theme that jumps out at me every time: most people believe THEIR pain isn't bad enough to warrant acknowledgement or treatment, so they invalidate their painful experiences.

If YOU think your life hasn't been "that bad," but you continue to eat or drink and sabotage your weight loss compulsively, then you've got some unmet needs, pain, or trauma.

Period.

It doesn't matter if someone had it worse than you.

You don't have to compare painful stories with anyone else.

Your pain is valid.

You deserve healing.

Yes, even *you*.

But I can tell you that all day long. If you don't find a way to believe it is true, you will stay stuck right here. You may be able to improve things here and there, but the next time you're "triggered," you'll be right back where you started.

I think at some point, for example, most of us figure out that sugar (or carbs or alcohol that break down into sugar) makes us feel better momentarily. Sugar is super addictive for a reason. It lights up the pleasure center in your brain, temporarily distracting you from the pain you're trying to escape.

Unfortunately, sugar also:

- Causes weight gain when consumed in excess.
- Leads to an increased risk of Type 2 diabetes, cancer, and heart disease
- Contributes to depression and anxiety.
- Causes increased hunger, cravings, inflammation, and fluid retention.

- Leads to nutrient deficiencies and high blood pressure.
- Causes headaches, migraines, and an increase in stress hormones.
- Disrupts the digestive system and sleep patterns.
- Interferes with the body's natural ability to repair itself.
- Leads to decreased concentration.
- Leads to weakened bones and increased fracture risk.
- Causes the skin to age prematurely.

So not only are you dealing with some painful experiences in your past, but you've become a sick, cranky, overweight, scatter-brained, older-looking version of yourself.

And if you're anything like me, you also blame yourself for your lack of willpower regarding the most addictive, readily available, socially acceptable drug on earth.

And by the way, if you're thinking, "Sugar isn't my issue," you're still not in the clear because *any* of your soft addictions light up that pleasure center of your brain, so they end up distracting you from your pain just like sugar.

Distraction doesn't heal your wound; it merely diverts your attention away from it.

These psychological and physiological responses are not your fault - it's human biology and unconscious conditioning. But we do have the ability to override these responses given the right tools.

And it begins with an awareness of the unconscious strategies that you've been using to deal with your pain.

A great example of me stumbling around in the dark before I

had Weighted Awareness was from one particular episode of WORKOUT, the Bravo TV show in which I co-starred as a celebrity trainer. I was talking to a fellow trainer, Doug Blasdell, on a hike after I had experienced yet another breakup. Doug was one of the sweetest people in the world who tragically passed away while we were shooting Season 2.

Doug asked me on camera, "If you weren't out here hiking right now, what would you be doing?"

And I answered, "I'd be at home, in bed, eating chocolate and watching some Jane Austin movie."

And, of course, after that hike, I felt better. But it didn't last.

What that episode DIDN'T show was what I did later that night: jumping into bed with my comfy pajamas and eating chocolate cake while watching Bridget Jones's Diary.

My hiking story pretty much sums up how I dealt with my feelings of sadness and disappointment before I knew better. I might be active during the day, but I would cocoon myself and eat comforting food while immersing myself in a comforting movie or book at night. The beneficial effects of that hike didn't outweigh my compulsion to soothe my heartache with the comfort I thought I needed.

I had unconsciously conditioned myself to self-sabotage habitually. Endorphins and willpower didn't have a chance at the end of the day.

I would eat to comfort myself – and because I liked exercise and had fitness friends, I would get out and do things, so I didn't think it was such a problem. After all, I still looked ok, and my weight didn't skyrocket. It would just kind of creep up a little here and a little there. I would really buckle down and do some extreme dieting and exercise, and that seemed to work… until it didn't.

I never asked myself WHY I felt the need to comfort myself with food. WHY was I in this cycle? WHY did I feel so compelled to have something sweet? WHY a whole pizza? WHY stay with this guy if he didn't treat me right? WHY did I always feel broke? WHY did I feel the need to retreat so much when everyone thought of me as a happy, successful, outgoing person?

The answer, I would later learn, is because I had unmet needs and painful experiences in my past that were never validated. In fact, I invalidated all my pain, telling myself it wasn't "that bad," and I kept denying the comfort my inner child sought.

I was unaware my inner child was upset about some past trauma. I barely knew who my inner child was, let alone that I was unconsciously invalidating her.

It took a long time for me to become aware of the relationship between validation and comfort-seeking coping mechanisms.

Guess what? In times of high stress or when you're particularly triggered, that part of your brain responsible for survival takes over, and you justify comfort any way you can.

So you'll just order the pizza because you tell yourself you don't have time to cook a healthy meal. You'll eat the chocolate because you tell yourself you "deserve a treat." You'll have some wine because you'll tell yourself you've had "a hard day." You'll stay in that relationship because you believe the fear of being alone is something you can't handle. You'll stick with that job you hate because at least there's a steady paycheck.

Oh, the things we tell ourselves to excuse our irresponsible behavior.

One minute, you're saying "F*ck it" to yourself (and the diet) while eating the whole pizza, then you're blaming yourself for not sticking to your diet.

Self-sabotage happens when we are unaware of what's going on in our minds.

You've likely already come to suspect that you will keep sabotaging your progress until you become aware of the underlying reasons why you seek comfort in food rather than working through the wounds that remain from needs that have never been met. To be clear, Step 1 is not about working through anything - it's about understanding that there IS SOMETHING that needs to be worked through, and without that awareness, we remain locked in a tug-o-war between "F*ck it" and self-blame.

The reason why we start here is that if we don't know what the problem is, if we don't acknowledge it - how can we ever begin to work through it?

We can't.

You may have been doing this dance for so long that your body is so inflamed or in physical pain, or depleted in nutrients that you struggle to see these symptoms for what they are. You're walking around with that fake smile, trying to convince yourself and everyone else that you're okay. But you're not.

You're not OK.

You are emotionally starving while physically overindulging. It's a coping mechanism that used to work if only temporarily, to make you feel better. Then it stopped working because the pain became bigger than a pizza could fix.

Where Do You Start?

You start with acknowledging your pain.

Maybe you got the silent treatment as a kid.

Maybe you were met with a defensive or dismissive parent when you tried to tell them how you felt.

Maybe other kids at school got things you wanted, but you never got.

Maybe someone criticized your body in some way.

Maybe someone looked at you or touched you in a way that made you feel unsafe or violated.

Maybe you endured physical punishments.

Maybe you were bullied by other kids or adults.

Maybe you felt abandoned.

Maybe you're still surrounded by a-holes.

Whatever made you feel pain… it's valid.

So validate it. Stop blowing it off, brushing it aside, pushing it down deep, or denying it even exists. Because let's face it, your old method of dealing with your pain hasn't worked – or you wouldn't be here.

Your foundation for healing and living an extraordinary life is built upon this crucial first step.

Take my client Alecia (name changed for her privacy), who identifies as being an overweight sugar addict and also a highly educated professional in the health and wellness industry. We used to laugh/cry about our sugar addictions together, so I thought I would reach out to see if she'd be interested in learning some of these techniques.

As a fellow intellectual skeptic, I knew it might be hard to break through the reasoning we typically use to justify our behavior, but she was willing to try this "new age-y woo woo" stuff, as she likes to call it.

I pointed out that thousands of successful studies showed that these neuroscience techniques helped with anxiety and depression… but not so many on weight loss. Since coping mechanisms like stress eating are a big part of anxiety, it seemed reasonable to connect the two.

After asking a few questions and digging into her connections between sugar and her emotional state, Alecia was surprised to remember that making cookies at Christmas time with her family suddenly popped up. Her mother had always been beauty-conscious and made her feel shameful for wanting to have treats – except at Christmas. She loved having her favorite aunts around with the entire family, and it was a joyous occasion where she was loved, accepted, and even encouraged to indulge.

Alecia realized that the pain of losing her aunts and the pain of not having unconditional acceptance from her mother other than at Christmas was why she loved all things sugar. With this new awareness, she could now see the connection between chocolate and self-soothing behavior.

When you get in touch with your pain, you can proceed with accepting it for what it is rather than smothering it in chocolate. Chocolate is great. Avoiding your pain isn't.

It's time to be brave.

STEP **2**

Weighted Acceptance

You've missed out on a lot.

It's natural to feel angry when you realize how much happiness has been robbed from you because you've been invalidating your pain for so long.

How might life have been different if you didn't have this pain in the first place?

What would your life be like if you didn't hide from opportunities because you didn't feel confident?

For example, I speak to many mothers who hide behind the camera. They don't feel like they look good enough, and they're embarrassed about their body – so they eat junk food and drink alcohol in a seemingly endless cycle of temporary comfort and shame.

I've also spoken to the adult children of mothers who hid from the camera - and you know what they regret? They did not have very many photos of their mom because she never felt good enough to be in a photo. And now she's gone – and she died sooner than she should have due to health complications.

Oof, right?

If only those women had understood their own emotional starvation, they may have been able to address it in time to do something about it. They could have accepted these "flaws" that they saw in themselves and worked to ensure their children would have happy memories of a strong, confident mother.

It's not their fault that they didn't have the resources or information that you now have.

We must learn to show ourselves some compassion for the child in us who didn't know better until she did.

So, what are you going to do now that you are aware?

I think a lot of moms feel stuck in their role as caregivers and mistake their self-harm for self-care. Distractions and unhealthy coping mechanisms that ultimately make you feel like hiding from the camera are NOT self-care - those are ways of escaping pain.

If you stay in that place where you know you've masked your pain in some way but try to convince yourself it wasn't that bad... you're not going to be as motivated to change. You've got to accept what your unhealthy coping mechanisms have robbed you of.

If you're having a hard time doing that, then here's a great exercise:

Imagine that you could go back in time to any age you wanted to be, and you had all the love, encouragement, confidence, time, and resources that you needed. No obstacles whatsoever...

What would you do with your life?

Who would you be?

How would life be different?

Some people have won the genetic lottery with inherent talent, good looks, loving caregivers, and financial advantages. However, I believe that two factors, time and energy, are required for success in any area of life.

If you put enough time and energy into learning a skill or nurturing a relationship, there's nothing you can't do.

That sounds simple until you factor in that your energy is easily depleted when you have unmet needs. The amount of time you focus your energy on dealing with mental or physical pain because of those unmet needs can add up to decades.

Those decades worth of distraction with unhealthy coping mechanisms have taken your energy away from what you want most out of life - whether it's great health, loving relationships, or career success.

So ask yourself - what have your distractions cost you?

Get in touch with accepting the pain of the opportunity cost of your unmet needs.

Did you not go for that career in something you love because you lacked confidence?

Did you miss out on the love of your life because you "didn't deserve" better?

Did you allow poor treatment from people around you because you were too scared to be on your own?

Did your health suffer because you were getting temporary hits of comfort?

If you really want to stay motivated, write down your answers.

Acceptance of what your coping mechanisms cost you (your time and energy!) is crucial. If you skip this step, you'll continue to mask your pain or convince yourself that your current situation is not that bad.

Or you'll waste more time wishing things had been different and resenting all the whys and hows.

The result is always the same - you're going to stay right where you are.

Do you agree with the philosophy that you are always in the right place at the right time, and whatever got you here is what you are supposed to be?

If you do, then believe that you were supposed to go through a bunch of pain to get to this point and take this as a sign that you're also supposed to be reading this book right now. You're supposed to learn this framework to finally neutralize a lifetime of unhealthy coping mechanisms.

I believe that no child deserves the pain they've had to endure, but it's up to them how they will deal with it when they're an adult.

For example, we can choose to learn from our pain and help others get through their pain quicker and easier by sharing our knowledge. That's what I'm choosing to do.

Once I finally accepted the consequences of my lack of awareness, I got angry about all the opportunities I missed out on. And how long it took me to get that awareness still makes me angry because time is our most precious resource.

Anger is a healthy response – and your body's way of sending you a message that your boundaries have been violated. There's a lot of power in anger but it's not healthy to stay there. Becoming a rage monster is not the goal. Anger is simply a signal that something needs to be changed.

So let's change it.

It's not your fault that you were unaware of your unmet needs. It's not your fault that you didn't know the consequences of your masked pain until now.

This step will allow you to get in touch with true desires after you've acknowledged the self-imposed obstacles that have gotten in your way.

But acceptance has two parts.

The first part is acknowledging the pain your coping strategies have cost you. It hurts. Taking a moment to feel that pain instead of distracting yourself from it is crucial to healing.

The second part is to accept life as it is – or love and support who you are right now – and that you're lucky enough to be alive, so you still have the chance to make changes.

So now that you are aware (Step 1) and now that you can accept who you are and the consequences of your unhealthy coping mechanisms (Step 2), you're ready to move on to the next step: WEIGHTLESS RESPONSIBILITY.

Responsibility is where you take back your power so you can navigate your vessel toward the life of your dreams.

Let's go, Cap'n!

STEP **3**

Weightless Responsibility

The Oxford Dictionary defines responsibility as follows:

re·spon·si·bil·i·ty
noun

> the state or fact of having a duty to deal with something or of having control over someone.

> "a true leader takes responsibility for their team and helps them achieve goals."

Taking responsibility has been preached to many of us since birth – yet very few know what it truly means to do so. It goes so far beyond just admitting when you're wrong, too.

One of the key moments in this step is when you realize that you have a duty to deal with your unmet needs and have control over your responses to whatever life dishes out to you. Think of it as response-ability – or the ability to respond to adversity or triggers in a more empowered or strategic way. This is the tough part, though.

But now that you've become aware of your unmet needs and accept what you've missed out on, it's finally POSSIBLE to change your responses. Without the prior two steps, you'd keep self-sabotaging yourself whenever you feel discomfort and never figure out why.

Taking responsibility for your responses FROM THIS POINT on is the key to improving your life. Because you didn't skip steps one and two, your past no longer equals your future.

It's not just about minimizing the number of times you get triggered, but it's about what you do after you get triggered – now that you know better.

It wasn't until I made the conscious effort to take time, energy, and resources to become aware of and validate my pain, then get in touch with the opportunity cost of remaining unaware for so long, that it became easier to replace unhealthy behaviors with better ones.

For example, turning off the TV binge-snacking session and getting more sleep became easier when I no longer unconsciously responded like a rebelling kid needing comfort. Now that I've validated my inner child's pain, she no longer demands an entire batch of chocolate chip cookies and a Harry Potter marathon or scrolling endlessly on social media.

This is not to say that those kinds of days aren't necessary or desirable once in a while.

But they shouldn't be a common occurrence as a countermeasure to adulting. Taking responsibility for how you handle those stressors is the gateway to unlocking that dream bod, that dream job, and that life you desire.

With better sleep, I finally started enjoying morning workouts (something I NEVER did). I also changed my focus to getting some sun to improve my mood, movement to release those "hope molecules" as a natural antidepressant, and techniques that made my back and knees feel better. I completely changed my workouts from being a punishment for guilty eating behaviors to an affirming feel-good session that's genuinely self-care.

Your subconscious mind dictates 80% of your behavior, and that is where your inner child resides. After you validate your inner child's pain, you no longer have a subconscious drive to seek comfort because you're already there! You've arrived at that place called peace.

Another way to think of how your subconscious mind affects your behavior is to imagine your mind as your computer with dozens of tabs open. If your computer runs all those programs in the background, the window you're working on (your conscious mind) will run slower. It won't be as efficient. But shut all those other programs down, and suddenly, life gets faster and easier.

It's the same way homemade chocolate chip cookies used to make me think of how I felt when I was younger. I once made a batch for myself and my friends at a sleepover. We were able to stay up all night. I felt loved and supported. I felt freedom and comfort. I felt great friendship without judgment.

Those cookies were also parental approval with a sugar rush — all of those feelings used to be wrapped up in my enjoyment of cookies.

Now, after acknowledging and comforting my inner child, I no longer crave them when I'm feeling stressed or lonely. They're just cookies. And I still really love the way they taste. But I can have just one and enjoy it instead of eating the whole batch because now the inner child residing in my subconscious mind is emotionally satiated.

At first, this may sound like a lot of hard work. But guess what? When you've gone through the first two steps and better understand why you chose your vices, where that behavior came from, and what those choices cost you, it suddenly won't seem unmanageable.

Believe it or not, after a while, alternative healthy coping mechanisms become not only easy but absolutely non-negotiable in your lifestyle.

It all starts with recognizing the fact that it's up to you to engrain these steps into your life until they become a habit. Sure, I can and will be there to support and motivate you to stick to them, but the real magic happens when these responses become second nature.

You soon realize that overindulging no longer feels necessary, and you are ready to undertake the things that help you strengthen your body, relationships, and confidence.

It takes courage to live an authentic, fulfilling life, and it's so much easier to have courage when you've healed those wounded parts of yourself you've been denying for so long.

If you skip the step where you validate your pain and you miss the stage where you accept how much it costs to invalidate your pain, you won't change your responses to triggers. Your escapism into unhealthy behaviors will continue when you feel like "no one is watching" – and that is depression, my friend.

Response-ability only occurs when you're healed enough to take a stand against those forces that have enslaved your potential. Taking responsibility for your new behaviors and habits is taking back your power from whatever or whoever took it from you.

You'll never know how powerful you are until you've gathered all that energy you've dispersed over the years, pointing your finger at anything or anyone but yourself.

Nothing can stop you once you take responsibility for your responses, behaviors, and habits.

But without taking responsibility, any actions you take to improve your life won't be effective or lasting. Aren't you tired of that not-so-merry-go-round?

And to be clear – you are NOT taking responsibility for any sh*t that was done to you.

Step 3 is taking responsibility for changing how you respond to situations going forward. Your response-ability will improve the more you flex that muscle, too.

Once you've built your foundations of awareness, acceptance, and responsibility, you're ready for the final and most crucial step – WEIGHTLESS INSPIRED ACTION!

STEP **4**

Weightless Inspired Action

In our house, we say wishes out loud, whether it's blowing out candles on a birthday cake or when we throw a coin in a fountain.

Whoever started the "keep wishes to yourself, or they won't come true" tradition was probably a skeptical, traumatized person tired of being let down by the world. When you voice your dreams out loud, they can become a reality.

If you keep all your wishes to yourself, how can anyone help you make them happen?

The truth is that you need people, and no one can do it all alone. Speaking your intentions into existence is where the magic begins, but where you go from there is up to you. Step 4 is where magic happens. And yes, I believe in magic – but not like when we were kids. It's not that magic words hold some special power; it's that words can INSPIRE ACTION.

In Step 1 of the Healthy Freedom Framework, we finally become aware of the fact that we're emotionally starving and have been for a very long time.

It's no wonder we've been overindulging.

In Step 2, we allowed ourselves to accept the good, the bad, and the ugly truth of our past so that we could move forward.

As we built that foundation, we then came to realize that it is our responsibility (Step 3) to reconcile our past with what's actually happening in the present and that, as adults, it's up to us to love and support ourselves, thereby fulfilling our own unmet needs from childhood. Then, we are able to respond to chaos and stress with healthier strategies.

Why is inspired action your next step? Because any other kind of action is unlikely to last.

On the other hand, an object at rest wants to remain at rest. It's why we find the couch so appealing when we're feeling down and out. It takes a big boost to get us going but less energy to KEEP us going.

Inspired Action means doing activities that heal you, strengthen you, energize you, and fill up your soul – rather than just provide a distraction from the pain.

Step 4 is the time to pinpoint which habits are going to be healthy for YOU.

Weightless Inspired Action is the jump-off point for the rest of our lives. We just have to make sure we're jumping in the right direction.

It certainly is easier to sit on the couch eating chips and watching Netflix than to dig into the "why" of your unhealthy coping behaviors – but it's much harder to deal with diabetes, heart attacks, failed relationships, and unfulfilled dreams, no?

Inspired action means to naturally let go of the coping mechanisms because there's nothing left to cope with. That is the payoff of working through Steps 1 through 3: you're not the same person.

It wasn't until I spoke out loud, "I have an idea for a gym," and my friend immediately said, "I love that. I'll invest in that idea." Exactly one year later, the doors to my award-winning elliptical studio opened after a ton of what I thought was inspired action.

Not so fast. When everything came crashing down in the wake of Covid, it felt like my world had fallen apart.

Clearly, my (inner) work was not done. I just didn't realize that my motivation was purely external.

The dream of my gym gave me a lot of motivation initially – but its failure made me feel like I wasn't enough. I had linked my value and happiness to a business venture's success.

That motivation didn't last because my unhealthy coping behaviors came right back when I was busy and stressed, and the outcome of a worldwide pandemic was out of my control. It wasn't until I took the time to dig deep into WHY I had those behaviors during the "bad" times that I healed many of my past unmet needs and adopted habits that made me feel confident, healthy, energized, and free.

I skipped steps one, two, and three when I opened the studio…

and that's why just cutting to the action step isn't enough.

If I had taken the time to go through all four steps before, I would have had a much different outcome. I didn't know any better. But now I do. And so do YOU!

Funny thing about the "bad" times, too… I've found that they can be the start of a beautiful new chapter, especially if you've taken the time to heal those unmet needs and see those unhealthy coping mechanisms just fall away.

Before I could take my business to the next level, I had to do the inner work.

There are no shortcuts.

Now, I get to coach people all over the world instead of just a couple-mile radius around the studio. It was because the studio closed that I was able to reach MORE people. Most businesses become a different version from where they started. They evolve. Your life is meant to change, too. You're meant to grow. You will try things and learn that it wasn't the best strategy… so you change it.

You learn and you keep going.

Why inspired ACTION? Because nothing will change unless you think and then do things differently. The first three steps all happen in your head. The last step involves you taking your healing and enlightened self – and changing your daily habits.

Your truly healed self simply doesn't need to consistently reach for unhealthy coping mechanisms.

It's no longer a battle of willpower.

That compulsion simply vanishes.

And when those unhealthy coping behaviors fall away, your ideal nutrition and activity is SOOOOO much easier to do and actually enjoy.

You might be thinking that there's no way you could feel confident, healthy, energized, and free by following the four steps I've described.

If you're like me, you've probably tried a bunch of ways to "get healthy" before and were let down by your results. You may have even had some success by working your tail off, and you're dreading having to do it once again.

But that's not working anymore, is it?

That's because it never was the answer... and you haven't tried *this* method.

I know you haven't tried it because you're still reading.

Wouldn't it be great if you could do all the things necessary to get back in alignment with your true, healed self while you optimize your food and fitness as quickly and painlessly as possible?

If you're nodding your head yes, then please... read on.

NEXT STEPS

It was Christmas morning in the Hollywood Hills, and I was completely happy eating Spaghettios in my apartment *alone.*

I didn't have enough money to fly home to Chicago to see my parents, and my brother's family in Long Beach wasn't getting together until later that day for dinner.

So, I had my first Christmas morning alone.

And it was amazing.

No family stress. No silent treatment because my Mom didn't like the present I gave her.

No yelling at me about doing something "the right way" or the day was ruined.

Nothing but glorious Chef Boyardee – and Scrooge dancing around singing, "Thank you very much!"

Weird, right? That should have been a wake-up call for me – but it wasn't. It took me about 20 more years to figure out that my dysfunctional family had some issues, which caused me a lifetime of self-doubt and emotional eating.

Don't let this be you. Twenty years is an excruciatingly long time that you can't get back.

If you're anything like the clients I've coached over the last few decades, the previous chapters have stirred up some emotion in you. And that's good! The last thing you want (or need) is to put this book down and forget how much pain you're carrying around. That's what your mind wants you to do: forget how much it hurts.

But what if, instead, you met the pain head-on and started healing the parts of you that have been begging for your attention instead of continuing to numb those painful emotions with more self-sabotaging behavior?

Those years you've spent feeling stuck, sick, and unhealthy have led you here, now, to a place where it all makes sense. There's no point in beating yourself up for *anything* anymore.

And shame has no place here.

Neither does self-doubt, that feeling of uncertainty where you question if it's even possible to change.

It is possible. At this point, all it takes is a decision to go through the process of eliminating those unhealthy habits and replacing them with empowering ones.

Shrug off that heavy weight that's been holding you down – and holding you back from becoming the best version of yourself.

To finally become the best version of yourself, to experience the best health, the greatest success, and the most nourishing relationships, you've got to let go of those behaviors that no longer serve you.

You can't finish the race with your feet firmly planted on the starting block, right? You've got to let go of your old way of doing things to gain a more empowered way of living.

And by the way, there is one place you can go to help you find awareness of your pain.

To gain acceptance of the consequences of your coping mechanisms.

Where you can improve your response-ability to those lifelong strategies that have kept you stuck.

And finally, get you into that authentic, empowered place where you feel confident, healthy, energized, and free.

My Healthy Freedom techniques, which pick up where we leave off with this book, are far more advanced than anything you may have tried in the past.

But – this is important for you to understand – advanced techniques will only work when you do.

This book has prepared you for advancement: to do the deeper work you've been missing. We've covered the steps that are almost always overlooked in all those diet books that promise you can "lose 7 pounds in 7 minutes" by telling you what to eat.

It would be like me sending you a meal plan, giving you a list of exercises, and saying, "Do this." It might work for a minute, but it wouldn't last. We both *know* that.

When people work with me, they are prepared to do the work. They already know it will work because I have set them up for success using my Healthy Freedom Formula. The more advanced techniques I use when I'm working directly with my clients are specifically designed to take what you've learned in this book and apply it to real-life circumstances, using a combination of proven mind/body strategies that provide lasting results.

What I've noticed with the people I've guided (and with myself, if I'm being honest) is that they have a lot of self-doubt at the beginning. It's understandable. We've spent years seeing weight and moods yo-yo and are super frustrated.

One woman in her mid-50s, Margaret (name has been changed), considered herself pretty successful in her business and felt relatively healthy – but she just couldn't seem to get her belly down. Nor could she seem to give up drinking several glasses of wine at social get-togethers and weeknights after a hard day at work.

She wanted me to just give her a diet and exercise plan initially, but I asked her if she'd be willing to try my Healthy Freedom Formula as a way to get a little deeper into her behavior patterns and reprogram her typical responses to stress and social triggers. She was a bit skeptical at first but was willing to try.

Margaret answered a few questions about her past experiences, and she shared that her father died when she was younger. She became the organizer of the family and even took care of meals for her older siblings (a lot of responsibility for a kid).

When Margaret got her first job out of school, she enjoyed drinking with co-workers and friends as a way to relax after work. She said it felt like freedom away from responsibility, and she could relax and be silly, too.

She was supposed to meet up with friends that weekend who loved to do winery trips together, so she was curious if my unique strategy could help. I walked her through my Healthy Freedom Formula to examine just one aspect of her behavior: drinking "too much" with friends. I wanted to see if she found any connections between her drinking behavior and past experiences and if we could transform her unconscious habit into something healthier.

Although Margaret seemed surprised, it was no surprise to me that she had quite a different outcome than she had been expecting just days before.

Not only did she NOT have the compulsion to drink, but she reported having felt a new level of clarity and authenticity when talking to her friends. And they all discussed that they, too, preferred not to wake up late, groggy and achy from drinking too much – and they ended up excited to get together more frequently with mocktail recipes and focus more on enjoying each other's company.

Since that weekend with her friends, Margaret has had other instances where she notices the comfort (and freedom) she associates with drinking wine – and we examine those, too. She is now on the right path because she is aware of her behavior and accepts the consequences alcohol has had in her life. She is learning to love who she is. She continues to improve her response-ability and reports feeling less stressed in situations that used to make her feel triggered.

Margaret still has a glass of wine here and there – but she no longer uses it as a coping mechanism for stress or as a means to connect with her friends. She realized that she no longer needed an "excuse to act silly" around her buddies and felt like she was embracing her true self more.

Margaret has also increased her muscle tone significantly and no longer has back aches because the nutrition and exercise plan I customized for her works so much better because she's not sabotaging her progress with excess wine and hangover comfort eating.

Perhaps you're wondering if you are so different from someone like Margaret that I couldn't possibly help you.

Well, let me ask you this using that knife analogy from before…

If you got sliced open with a knife, you'd probably be distracted by the pain, right? Your focus would be to stop that pain and you'd be putting energy into that solution. You'd get your shot of morphine to numb the pain - but that wound would still be there. And what if every time you even thought about that wound, it got sliced open all over again?

And a shot of morphine doesn't numb the pain forever, right? Only for a little while.

Then, you'd still have to take the time, energy, and money to get more morphine. Meanwhile, you're missing work or friend get-togethers or date night because you're busy trying to numb that wound – but it's not actually healed, so this pain/morphine cycle keeps repeating itself over years and years. Plus, you've lived a long time so now every time ANY knife is seen or referenced in your life, it feels like another wound, so it takes more and more energy to deal with it.

Now imagine that I've shown you the disinfectant, the bandage, and the healing process for closing that wound once and for all... but you don't DO anything about it. Wouldn't that be silly?

No one can change what has happened in your life. But we CAN change how you process and RESPOND to that memory. So yes, I can help you.

Here's the thing that all therapists and doctors agree on when it comes to the mental and emotional wounds that affect our body: it's the meaning that we give an event that affects us. It's the meaning that has us reaching for a coping mechanism... or not.

And we can absolutely reframe the meaning of events in our lives given the right tools and support.

Everything works so much better when you're in alignment with your truly healed self, and that only happens when you've adjusted the meanings of events that used to disempower you. You're able to respond to situations with healthier strategies when you know the why behind the how.

So you've got three options at this point.

1. You can do nothing and live as if it's "not so bad" even though your health and life are suffering.
2. You can do it alone, buying more books and going on YouTube, spending HOURS and HOURS of time doing research and spending years testing out healing modalities that may or may not work, along with

diets and workouts that continue to frustrate you or even injure you.

3. OR... You can hire someone who can get you there a lot faster (as in years and years faster) without the confusion, stress, and despair that comes with trying to do it yourself.

The next logical step would be to work with someone, don't you think? If you think about it, time is our most precious resource. We can't ever get it back. And make no mistake, getting this done fast is LIFE-changing.

I used to be one of those people who would say, "I don't have the time" (or the money) when it came to investing in myself until I heard someone say, "If I gave you $100,000,000 today, would you take it?"

"Of course I would!"

"Would you still take it if I said you could have it – but you wouldn't wake up tomorrow?"

"Wow. No."

"Then why are you waking up every day acting like your life isn't worth $100,000,000?"

OMG, right?

Your life is so precious. Your time is EVERYTHING. Don't waste more time dealing with habits and old wounds that can be healed much faster than you can imagine.

You've been weighted down long enough.

If you're still not sure about what to do next, head on over to my website and check out the quiz I made to help you figure out exactly what to do next at www.ZenBurgos.com.

If nothing else, I promise you'll know exactly how much "weight" you've been carrying around.

I've been where you are right now… struggling and searching for a healthier way of meeting life's challenges with a more energized, authentic, and empowered version of myself. I stumbled for so long, and I wished that someone could have held my hand through this process decades ago, but it was not available until I put all the necessary ingredients together. I feel so much more alive and peaceful, yet excited about the future now.

There is hope.

I invite you to reach out for guidance so you can soon meet the best version of yourself, too.

Whatever you decide to do at this moment, I wish you the best of luck on your journey!

But one last word of advice: do not close this book and reach out for that same old comfort blanket.

If you've read this far, some part of you wants change.

You know where to find me!

ACKNOWLEDGMENTS

There are so many people I'd like to thank for making this book possible.

To my husband, David, thank you for allowing me the freedom to explore my mind, my heart, and my health. Without your love and support, this book would not have been possible.

To my daughter, Chariot, who has shown me what unconditional love is… thank you for being the wonderful person you are. Being your mommy is the greatest gift and bestest thing in the whole world.

To my best friend, Jen, thank you for all the times we've laughed and cried through this roller coaster we've been living. Your joyful radiance, understanding, and loyalty are such a treasure.

To Magic and Larissa, thank you for all your love and support when I needed it most.

Many thanks also go out to:

All my clients who've become good friends and shared their fitness journeys with me.

All those outstanding and supportive members and staff of The HIT Locker and ELLIPTIHIT.

Lin, Dustin, Rhianon and my fellow writers Laura, Tunisha, Sandy, Jennifer, Dawn, Tracy, and Connie who have helped me so much with tweaking specific phrases and helped me bring this labor of love to light.

Tina, Christina, and Megan for helping me process grief and rage and embrace more self-love.

The magical people at Soderworld, my sanctuary away from home.

My lovely neighborhood of Brook Crossing that exemplifies a wonderful spirit of community.

Cathy, Naomi, Amber, and The Branch community of women that have inspired me and encouraged me, and embraced me as the sweat-pant-loving mom that I am.

Amanda and my fellow entrepreneurs, thank you for the great read and those Monday night chats.

The amazing women who've shared their complicated and emotional health and wellness stories with me.

All the people I've had the opportunity to work with in my life, whether to lead or follow your lead, my sincere thanks.

My brother, Trey, for the fond memories of blither, mix tapes, thoughtful birthday gifts, making me a first-time aunt to your awesome kids, and for helping me so much after foot surgery.

My sister, for helping me through the toughest part of my life the best she could.

My parents, for doing their best with their own unhealed trauma and teaching me lessons I never wanted to learn.

ABOUT THE AUTHOR

Zen Burgos is a lifelong learner when it comes to all things health-related and has over 30 years of experience in the fitness, nutrition, and motivational psychology world.

Best known as a celebrity trainer and stand-up comic from Bravo's TV show WORKOUT, Zen enjoys blending her fitness and weight loss tips in a humorous and non-judgy way. She acknowledges that trauma and unmet needs are NOT hilarious topics but necessary to explore when dealing with totally understandable stress-eating issues.

Zen is currently studying to get her Masters in Positive Psychology. She enjoys expanding her veggie garden, dabbling in Feng Shui, and going for nature walks with her husband, daughter, and dogs.

You can learn more about Zen's sabotage reversal weight loss coaching at www.zenburgos.com, or if you have questions, you can shoot her an email at zen@zenburgos.com Her award-winning elliptical and strength workout, ELLIPTIHIT, can also be accessed in the app store by anyone worldwide with a phone and bad knees.

Weighted
By Zen Burgos
www.ZenBurgos.com

Published by AFGO Press
AFGOpress.com

Made in the USA
Monee, IL
14 October 2023